M000093058

THIS BIRTH REGISTER BELONGS TO:

....

....

A OWN notebooks PRODUCTION

It is recommended that you use non-identifiable details in order to respect your client's confidentiality, and also to keep this book in a secure place. Please gain consent when entering details in to this book where you feel a person could be identified.

Birth Number	Date & Time	Parity	Type of Birth	Location	Baby Gender

Condition of Perineum	Third Stage	Complications	Pregnancy Notes

Birth Number	Date & Time	Parity	Type of Birth	Location	Baby Gender

Condition of Perineum	Third Stage	Complications	Pregnancy Notes

Birth Number	Date & Time	Parity	Type of Birth	Location	Baby Gender

Condition of Perineum	Third Stage	Complications	Pregnancy Notes

Birth Number	Date & Time	Parity	Type of Birth	Location	Baby Gender

Condition of Perineum	Third Stage	Complications	Pregnancy Notes

Birth Number	Date & Time	Parity	Type of Birth	Location	Baby Gender

Condition of Perineum	Third Stage	Complications	Pregnancy Notes

Birth Number	Date & Time	Parity	Type of Birth	Location	Baby Gender

Condition of Perineum	Third Stage	Complications	Pregnancy Notes

Birth Number	Date & Time	Parity	Type of Birth	Location	Baby Gender

Condition of Perineum	Third Stage	Complications	Pregnancy Notes

Birth Number	Date & Time	Parity	Type of Birth	Location	Baby Gender

Condition of Perineum	Third Stage	Complications	Pregnancy Notes

Birth Number	Date & Time	Parity	Type of Birth	Location	Baby Gender

Condition of Perineum	Third Stage	Complications	Pregnancy Notes

Birth Number	Date & Time	Parity	Type of Birth	Location	Baby Gender

Condition of Perineum	Third Stage	Complications	Pregnancy Notes

Birth Number	Date & Time	Parity	Type of Birth	Location	Baby Gender

Condition of Perineum	Third Stage	Complications	Pregnancy Notes

Birth Number	Date & Time	Parity	Type of Birth	Location	Baby Gender

Condition of Perineum	Third Stage	Complications	Pregnancy Notes

Birth Number	Date & Time	Parity	Type of Birth	Location	Baby Gender

Condition of Perineum	Third Stage	Complications	Pregnancy Notes

Birth Number	Date & Time	Parity	Type of Birth	Location	Baby Gender

Condition of Perineum	Third Stage	Complications	Pregnancy Notes

Birth Number	Date & Time	Parity	Type of Birth	Location	Baby Gender

Condition of Perineum	Third Stage	Complications	Pregnancy Notes

Birth Number	Date & Time	Parity	Type of Birth	Location	Baby Gender

Condition of Perineum	Third Stage	Complications	Pregnancy Notes

Birth Number	Date & Time	Parity	Type of Birth	Location	Baby Gender

Condition of Perineum	Third Stage	Complications	Pregnancy Notes

Birth Number	Date & Time	Parity	Type of Birth	Location	Baby Gender

Condition of Perineum	Third Stage	Complications	Pregnancy Notes

Birth Number	Date & Time	Parity	Type of Birth	Location	Baby Gender

Condition of Perineum	Third Stage	Complications	Pregnancy Notes

Birth Number	Date & Time	Parity	Type of Birth	Location	Baby Gender

Condition of Perineum	Third Stage	Complications	Pregnancy Notes

Birth Number	Date & Time	Parity	Type of Birth	Location	Baby Gender

Condition of Perineum	Third Stage	Complications	Pregnancy Notes

Birth Number	Date & Time	Parity	Type of Birth	Location	Baby Gender

Condition of Perineum	Third Stage	Complications	Pregnancy Notes

Birth Number	Date & Time	Parity	Type of Birth	Location	Baby Gender

Condition of Perineum	Third Stage	Complications	Pregnancy Notes

Birth Number	Date & Time	Parity	Type of Birth	Location	Baby Gender

Condition of Perineum	Third Stage	Complications	Pregnancy Notes

Birth Number	Date & Time	Parity	Type of Birth	Location	Baby Gender

Condition of Perineum	Third Stage	Complications	Pregnancy Notes

Birth Number	Date & Time	Parity	Type of Birth	Location	Baby Gender

Condition of Perineum	Third Stage	Complications	Pregnancy Notes

Birth Number	Date & Time	Parity	Type of Birth	Location	Baby Gender

Condition of Perineum	Third Stage	Complications	Pregnancy Notes

Birth Number	Date & Time	Parity	Type of Birth	Location	Baby Gender

Condition of Perineum	Third Stage	Complications	Pregnancy Notes

Birth Number	Date & Time	Parity	Type of Birth	Location	Baby Gender

Condition of Perineum	Third Stage	Complications	Pregnancy Notes

Birth Number	Date & Time	Parity	Type of Birth	Location	Baby Gender

Condition of Perineum	Third Stage	Complications	Pregnancy Notes

Birth Number	Date & Time	Parity	Type of Birth	Location	Baby Gender

Condition of Perineum	Third Stage	Complications	Pregnancy Notes

Birth Number	Date & Time	Parity	Type of Birth	Location	Baby Gender

Condition of Perineum	Third Stage	Complications	Pregnancy Notes

Birth Number	Date & Time	Parity	Type of Birth	Location	Baby Gender

Condition of Perineum	Third Stage	Complications	Pregnancy Notes

Birth Number	Date & Time	Parity	Type of Birth	Location	Baby Gender

Condition of Perineum	Third Stage	Complications	Pregnancy Notes

Birth Number	Date & Time	Parity	Type of Birth	Location	Baby Gender

Condition of Perineum	Third Stage	Complications	Pregnancy Notes

Birth Number	Date & Time	Parity	Type of Birth	Location	Baby Gender

Condition of Perineum	Third Stage	Complications	Pregnancy Notes

Birth Number	Date & Time	Parity	Type of Birth	Location	Baby Gender

Condition of Perineum	Third Stage	Complications	Pregnancy Notes

Birth Number	Date & Time	Parity	Type of Birth	Location	Baby Gender

Condition of Perineum	Third Stage	Complications	Pregnancy Notes

Birth Number	Date & Time	Parity	Type of Birth	Location	Baby Gender

Condition of Perineum	Third Stage	Complications	Pregnancy Notes

Birth Number	Date & Time	Parity	Type of Birth	Location	Baby Gender

Condition of Perineum	Third Stage	Complications	Pregnancy Notes

Birth Number	Date & Time	Parity	Type of Birth	Location	Baby Gender

Condition of Perineum	Third Stage	Complications	Pregnancy Notes

Birth Number	Date & Time	Parity	Type of Birth	Location	Baby Gender

Condition of Perineum	Third Stage	Complications	Pregnancy Notes

Birth Number	Date & Time	Parity	Type of Birth	Location	Baby Gender

Condition of Perineum	Third Stage	Complications	Pregnancy Notes

Birth Number	Date & Time	Parity	Type of Birth	Location	Baby Gender

Condition of Perineum	Third Stage	Complications	Pregnancy Notes

Birth Number	Date & Time	Parity	Type of Birth	Location	Baby Gender

Condition of Perineum	Third Stage	Complications	Pregnancy Notes

Birth Number	Date & Time	Parity	Type of Birth	Location	Baby Gender

Condition of Perineum	Third Stage	Complications	Pregnancy Notes

Birth Number	Date & Time	Parity	Type of Birth	Location	Baby Gender

Condition of Perineum	Third Stage	Complications	Pregnancy Notes

Birth Number	Date & Time	Parity	Type of Birth	Location	Baby Gender

Condition of Perineum	Third Stage	Complications	Pregnancy Notes

Birth Number	Date & Time	Parity	Type of Birth	Location	Baby Gender

Condition of Perineum	Third Stage	Complications	Pregnancy Notes

Birth Number	Date & Time	Parity	Type of Birth	Location	Baby Gender

Condition of Perineum	Third Stage	Complications	Pregnancy Notes

Birth Number	Date & Time	Parity	Type of Birth	Location	Baby Gender

Condition of Perineum	Third Stage	Complications	Pregnancy Notes

Birth Number	Date & Time	Parity	Type of Birth	Location	Baby Gender

Condition of Perineum	Third Stage	Complications	Pregnancy Notes

Birth Number	Date & Time	Parity	Type of Birth	Location	Baby Gender

Condition of Perineum	Third Stage	Complications	Pregnancy Notes

Birth Number	Date & Time	Parity	Type of Birth	Location	Baby Gender

Condition of Perineum	Third Stage	Complications	Pregnancy Notes

Birth Number	Date & Time	Parity	Type of Birth	Location	Baby Gender

Condition of Perineum	Third Stage	Complications	Pregnancy Notes

Birth Number	Date & Time	Parity	Type of Birth	Location	Baby Gender

Condition of Perineum	Third Stage	Complications	Pregnancy Notes

Birth Number	Date & Time	Parity	Type of Birth	Location	Baby Gender

Condition of Perineum	Third Stage	Complications	Pregnancy Notes

11771408R00066

Made in the USA
Monee, IL
16 September 2019